Made in the USA
Monee, IL
19 October 2020

45545606R00056